Self Esteem For Women

The #1 Self Esteem Guide For Women

I0419459

Mia Conrad

STOP!!! Before you read any further....Would you like to know the Secrets of Transforming your life, overcome insecurities, develop leadership skills, and undeniable confidence in your personal, professional, and relationship life?

If your answer is yes, then you are not alone. Thousands of people are looking for the secret to have unstoppable confidence and self-driven power in all areas of their lives.

If you have been searching for these answers without much luck, you're in the right place!

Not only will you gain incredible insight in this book, but because I want to make sure to give you as much value as possible, right now for a limited time you can get full **100% FREE access to a VIP bonus EBook** entitled **LIMITLESS ENERGY!**

Just Go Here For Free Instant Access:

www.PotentialRise.com

Legal Notice

Disclaimer Notice

information contained herein on the new conditions whenever they see applicable.

Table Of Contents

Introduction

Chapter 1 - Understand The Source Of Self Esteem

Chapter 2 - Change Your Inner Voice

Chapter 3 - Nourish Yourself

Chapter 4 - Make Your Surroundings Matter

Conclusion

Preview Of: "Happiness: *Secrets From The Happiest People On Earth*"

Free Bonus Offer

Introduction

I want to thank you and congratulate you for purchasing the book, *"Self Esteem For Women - The #1 Self Esteem Guide For Women"*.

This book contains proven steps and strategies on how to help you improve your self esteem and bring out the best in you. In the process, you will get to know more about yourself and your surroundings. All in all, this will be an enriching journey for you.

It is natural for a person to have wavering emotions and thoughts regarding themselves based on what is happening in their lives. Your work environment, your social life, and your relationships with loved ones all affect you.

Your self esteem, on the other hand, is much more important than any happenings in your life. Regardless as to whether you are going through the highs or lows in your life, your self esteem is the one that will influence how you react to these changes. A healthy self esteem will give you the confidence to face life's challenges; a low self esteem will make you feel worn out.

Oftentimes, a woman who has self esteem issues would be constantly burdened by the lows in her life. She has a lot of anxieties that negatively affect how she goes about her day.

A woman who has a healthy sense of self is someone who is able to take a step back and assess their feelings and situation in an objective manner, not letting any lows overwhelm them or any highs makes them feel superior. Healthy self esteem means that you value yourself and accept yourself for who you are. They are able to recognize their strengths and use these to their advantage, as well as understand their weaknesses but do not let these define who they are.

The main purpose of this book is to help you boost your self esteem so that you will be able to realize that you are a wonderful woman of the world who can live her life to the fullest. Keep in mind that nourishing your self esteem will take time, and this will require a promise from you to be open and to commit to making changes in your life.

Thanks again for purchasing this book, I hope you enjoy it!

Chapter 1 - Understand The Source Of Self Esteem

Before learning how to improve your self esteem, it is best to know where it comes from. First of all, self esteem is that feeling of pride for yourself; too much of it and you will be annoying, but self esteem that is too low will keep you from getting the best out of life.

Confidence should not be mistaken as self esteem. When you are confident, you feel comfortable, even joyous, when you are on stage in front of an applauding audience. A model, actor, and public speaker can be very confident when they are in front of a crowd. However, they could still have low self esteem once they go to the back stage.

Self esteem is all about whether you like yourself, whether you think that you deserve happiness and love. It is the driving force inside your mind that tells you how to live your life and deal with difficulties.

Self esteem continues to develop throughout life as we continue to experience new things and interact with different people. As a matter of fact, your childhood experiences made a big impact on your self esteem now. How other children socialized with you, how the adults treated you, and your accomplishments and the praise that you get from them all play a role.

The little girl that was praised, loved, and given attention to by her peers is usually the one who grows up to have healthy self esteem. Unfortunately, the little girl who was criticized and made fun of is the one who grows up to be a woman who has love self esteem. It is sad to think that the latter would sound more familiar to you.

Now that you are a grown woman, reflect on how you feel about yourself and the people around you. Do you feel loved and liked? Can you easily gain friends, find solutions to problems, and figure out ways on how to reach your goals? A woman with healthy self esteem will immediately say yes to these questions, and, yes, so can you!

Self esteem directly affects all aspects of your life. It will have an effect on your school and work performances, build networks, gain friends, establish romantic relationships, and altogether your physical, emotional, and psychological wellbeing. How you make your decisions is affected by your self esteem, along with how you deal with failures and letdowns.

Keep in mind that you will have to exert effort to boost your self esteem, but this challenge will give you results that will benefit you for the rest of your life.

How to Tell if You have Low Self Esteem

A woman with low self esteem is unable to be assertive even if she knows that she is doing what is right. She is not happy with her body image and often compares herself with others. She feels anxious whenever she meets other people, and is unable to talk about herself in a positive light such as telling others about her achievements and good qualities. She also finds it hard to accept compliments from others.

She does not know how to balance the different aspects of her life, and often feels burned out. She finds it difficult to maintain a healthy, solid relationship with others and would often feel anxious at the thought of them leaving her for someone who is "better." She does not feel satisfied with how she is living her life and finds it difficult or impossible to get out of her situation. She feels unworthy of anything and sometimes goes out of her way to please people because she is scared of being rejected. She often feels depressed and/or bitter towards others and is easily affected by the tribulations in her life.

Oftentimes, women with low self esteem tend to settle with what they have, but it is a different kind of acceptance from being happy about oneself. Instead, it is her thinking that she is simply a product of her past and she should just grit her teeth and bear with her unhappiness because that is just the way it will be for her life.

Women with low self esteem have the tendency to turn to alcoholism, drugs, nymphomania, or will develop psychological disorders if the self esteem issues are left unaddressed.

If you have said yes to most of these statements after reading them, then you should give yourself a pat on the back for doing something about your self esteem now. You are already taking action to making a positive change in your life, and the next chapters will guide you on your way to becoming a more confident woman who is happy and proud of herself.

Chapter 2 - Change Your Inner Voice

Dwelling on the past or simply submitting yourself to the status quo can damage your life now and in the future. How you see yourself is far more important than how other people see you. Throughout your entire life, you are your own true companion, 100 percent. Nobody else can be you, and you cannot be anybody else.

If you have low self esteem, your inner voice may not be very friendly right now. This inner voice is harsh, cold, and judgmental. However, you have the power to change "her" and turn her into your best friend. You can develop the inner voice of those women who have wonderfully healthy self esteem. Their inner voice is calm, kind, confident, and positive.

To change your inner voice, you must learn how to counteract her. Right now, your inner voice will still be the sad, bitter being inside your mind who finds something negative to say about everything that you do. Only this time, whenever you start to hear her, you immediately counteract it by saying something positive. Whenever she says that you did something poorly, say that you can always do better. Instead of letting her tell you that you are too fat or skinny, aim to live more healthily instead of feeling bad about how your body looks. If she says that you can't do it, fight back and say yes! Of course I can! If they can do it, so can I.

Develop the habit of positive affirmation, and your inner voice will gradually change her ways and become the reassuring and supportive best friend that you want her to be.

Positive affirmations are a form of positive therapy wherein you submit yourself an environment that quells the negativity in your mind. It is a powerful strategy to boost your self esteem and free you from being too reliant on the opinions of others about you.

Use the Power of Music

Listen to empowering music in the morning to boost your energy and get you revved up for the day. Likewise, listen to soothing music before you go to bed at night so that your mind will feel rested. Choose songs that make you feel good about yourself and appreciative of your life. Let the lyrics sink into your mind.

You can also play energetic and relaxing instrumental music while at the same time read positive, inspirational, and motivating passages that will help you to change how your inner voice works.

Develop a Healthy and Fixed Routine

To make positive affirmation work for you, start an invigorating morning routine and a relaxing night routine. When your body is constantly tired, your mind starts to feel stressed out and this can have an effect on your self esteem. A well rested mind often has room for happy thoughts. Set a specific time for when you go to bed and wake up in the morning, but make sure that you will get to sleep at least 7 hours every day.

When you wake up in the morning, follow a routine that will enable you to reflect on thoughts, plan your day, get you moving in the form of exercise, and nourish your body by eating a healthy breakfast.

Before you go to bed, reward yourself with a bubble bath or a warm shower, and then drink a hot cup of tea while writing all of your worries and anticipations of the next day in the journal to clear your mind for sleep.

Be vigilant in establishing a routine, for studies show that most happy and successful people are those who get enough sleep and wake up early to exercise and prepare for their days ahead. That's partially because they feel that they are in control of their lives when they follow a routine. Think of it this way: your inner voice will be a lot nicer if you are well-rested and in charge of your schedule.

Create a Mantra

To drown out the negativity coming from your inner voice, recite a mantra that will give you positive affirmation. These are in the form of short sentences filled with words of encouragement and praise that start with "I am" and "I can".

With "I am", you continue with positive adjectives that you would like to describe about yourself. For instance, you can say: "I am strong", "I am smart", "I am beautiful", "I am brave", "I am kind." What matters is that you say it every day, whether or not your inner voice tells you that it is true. The more you say it, the more truthful it will become.

Likewise, with "I can", follow with actions that you would like to accomplish in your life. For example, "I can have healthy self esteem", "I can make friends", "I can live a healthy lifestyle", "I can wake up early", "I can fight for myself", "I can do even better."

Make these mantras a part of your life by reciting them every day. You can even create visuals of them to remind you. For instance, you can print and post a piece of paper that says: "I am unique and beautiful" on a spot where you can instantly see it after you wake up in the morning. You can also post some more in other parts of your house or office, such as your mirrors, your work desk, your wallet, and as a desktop background of your computer. Be as creative as you can in making positive affirmations a part of your life.

Chapter 3 - Nourish Yourself

One powerful way to boost your self esteem is to seek self-improvement. Many individuals who have low self esteem dwell on their past failures, mistakes, and comparing themselves to others without doing anything about it. It is a comfort zone that is preventing them from growing.

When you take good care of yourself, you are also affirming that you love yourself and that you are worth the time and effort to improve. Self esteem grows as you continue to work on your way to seeing and feeling great. Yes, it will take effort, but it is very much worth it.

Take Care of Your Body

Many women have body image issues because they compare themselves too much with models on magazines, runways, and celebrities who can afford to pay for high end personal trainers. Instead of looking at other women who have been working hard on their bodies and feeling bad about yours, focus instead on making your body healthy and fit.

Everyone comes in different shapes and sizes, and your results can be different from your best friends' results, so comparing will not do you any good. Plan a regular exercise routine; something as simple as jogging every five thirty in the morning will do wonders to your body and soul. Watch free online videos that will teach you different exercises in your home so that you do not have to go to the gym. Have a workout buddy and encourage each other to keep going. Most of all, be persistent. Do not obsess over the results, but pay particular attention to your commitment.

Taking care of yourself also includes eating the right foods. Certain foods actually make you feel sluggish and contribute to your feelings of depression and anxiety. Research and ask a nutritionist about the certain types of food you should eat to make you healthier and feel better. There are tons of recipes online that you can use to whip up a quick and nutritious meal. Promise yourself that you are going to start feeding your body healthier meals and you will certainly start feeling better about yourself.

Remember to take a break every now and then as well. Take a nap if you need to, eat a piece of dark chocolate if you are craving for something sweet, watch a chick flick, and other little ways for your to de-stress. Do not be guilty of getting a manicure at a salon every now and then; seeing how clean and polished your nails are will instantly make you feel better.

Speaking of which, being fashionable will also do wonders to your self esteem. You do not have to spend a lot on signature clothes. Look for clever ways on how to dress for your body type and get the clothes that fit the description. When you see yourself so put together on the mirror, it will make you feel happy about the way you look and more confident in dealing with others. The simple rule of thumb for women is to always have a little black dress, killer high heels, a corporate jacket and pencil skirt, and of course, sexy lingerie in her closet.

Immerse Yourself in Something New

When a person discovers a hidden talent or hobby, she feels a sense of purpose. Seek to learn new things about yourself and about something that interests you. Remind yourself of what your strengths and abilities. It might seem difficult at first, particularly if you have low self esteem, but give it a try.

Sit down with a pen and paper and write down everything that you like about yourself. You can also keep all of your accomplishments in one clear book - your awards, certificates, and everything else that makes you feel good about being you. Knowing that you have come so far will encourage you to strive for more.

Then, think of something new that you would like to learn. It could be learning a different language, engaging in a sport, taking an online course, starting a garden, or crocheting... anything that will make your mind work and keep you interested. If it does not work out, don't fret. Reward yourself for having tried it. If it works out, then great! Just remember that it is okay to make mistakes as well, because you are learning.

Learning something new is a great way to boost your skills. Knowing that you are good at something will make you feel a better sense of self worth.

Chapter 4 - Make Your Surroundings Matter

Your relationships and your environment play a critical role in the development of your self esteem. Take a step back and think about what you currently have that are good or bad to your growth as a person.

Seek Support from the People Who Matter

You do not have to go through this journey alone. It is important to have the right people encourage you and back you up. You deserve all the help that you can get from supportive and positive friends and family.

Getting support from others would mean letting go of relationships that put you down. This is a vital but challenging part of growing. You have to say goodbye to the people who make you feel bad about yourself. You do not need them in your life. You can gently tell them that it makes you feel bad when they say bad things about you, and see if they will change. If not, then it is time to let go.

Don't be afraid to ask help from your friends. Tell them that you are working on how to improve yourself and you can all have a little activity where you ask each other what you like about each other. Hearing good things about yourself from a friend will certainly make you feel much better about yourself.

Find a mentor who can guide you through challenging times in work or school as well. You do not have to go through a difficult project alone, and then feel bad about yourself if you think that you are not doing well. Your supervisor or professor will be more than happy to help guide you through your learning experience and give you advice. They will respect you for making an effort.

Create a Positive Environment

Your surroundings, from the people you interact with everyday to your environment, all contribute to your level of self esteem. Waking up to a cluttered bedroom, for instance, will immediately make you think of chaos.

The essential trait of a positive environment is that it should be a place of comfort and encouragement. If your clutter is making you feel that way, then there are no changes needed. However, if it makes you feel bad about yourself, then take the time to get up and do something about it.

You can ask help from someone to throw away the old things that you no longer need. Change the colors of the walls to something more cheery, if you can. Install wall decals or hang up pictures of images and words that make you feel strong and happy. By making your environment more liveable and cozy, your mind will start to work better in bringing out your full potential. After all, there are better things to do than spending too much time searching for something missing from a pile of stuff.

In terms of your relationships, the key is communication. A positive environment is a place where your friends and family accept, understand, and encourage each other. One's efforts and accomplishments are recognized, and no room is given for criticism.

When one makes a mistake, constructive feedback and words of encouragement are given instead. There is no manipulation and abuse, but there is freedom of self-expression. And there is plenty of time for showing affection and bonding. Find ways for your loved ones to live harmoniously with each other. It might simply be a one heart-to-heart talk away. Aim to have at least one meal together each day.

And if you family is not the kind that will cooperate no matter what, then become a part of a community that does. Remember that there will always be people who might want to stir the pot and create bad vibes, but how you feel inside is within your control.

Take everything as a learning experience and do not let anything stop you from growing into a better and happy woman. You are certainly worth it.

Conclusion

Thank you again for purchasing this book on self esteem for women!

I am extremely excited to pass this information along to you, and I am so happy that you now have read and can hopefully implement these strategies going forward.

I hope this book was able to help you understand how to improve your self esteem and how to accomplish what you want in this life.

The next step is to get started using this information and to hopefully live a happier, healthier and much more fulfilling life!

If you know of anyone else that could benefit from the information presented here please inform them of this book.

Finally, if you enjoyed this book and feel it has added value to your life in any way, please take the time to share your thoughts and post a review on Amazon. It'd be greatly appreciated!

Thank you and good I wish you the best of luck!

Preview Of:

<u>Happiness</u>

Secrets From The Happiest People On Earth

Introduction

I want to thank you and congratulate you for purchasing the book **Happiness:** *Secrets From The Happiest People On Earth*. This book contains information about the Happiest People on Earth, as well as, insights on how you can apply these same principles to your life!

If you want to be happy, you have to first ask yourself what it is that's making you feel blue. Before you trek the path that will help you solve your issues, you have to be totally rid of conflict with who you are. If the kind of happy you want to experience is unadulterated, being honest with yourself is the starting point.

Are you down because you're discontented with your position in life? Has your partner left you? Have you moved to another city and haven't coped with the changes yet? Do you think that the number of friends you have isn't enough? Or are you still grieving the death of a family member?

For whatever reason it is, you have to admit that being sad bites. Seeing the world in a gloomy perspective is tough. Rather than continue with your ways, consider giving yourself a break. Way too many times, it has been said that life is short. So why waste moments being stuck in a downward spiral?

Here are 15 of the happiest people on earth. From social workers, artists, and businessmen to athletes and musicians, you can get some much-needed tips. Taking a peek at their situations in life may just open your eyes to what you deem to be the problem in yours.

Thanks again for purchasing this book. I hope you enjoy it!

Chapter 1 – The Joy In Social Work

"True happiness comes from the joy of deeds well done, the zest of creating things new." -Antoine de Saint-Exupery

Social workers are among the happiest on earth because they know that by doing another a favor, they are doing themselves a much bigger favor. They aren't oblivious to the fact that the rewards of making people's day are incomparable. These people are happy because they have made way for others to smile. Like them, if you're desperate for some mood-lifting, try clearing your schedule, be spontaneous, and cheer someone up. In your own way, you should take steps to change the world too.

Happy Person #1: Desmond Tutu

As a South African social rights activist, Desmond Tutu rose to fame. He helped his fellowmen by fighting against AIDS, poverty, racism, and sexism. He also opposed the Apartheid revolution and won the 1984 Nobel Peace Prize for it. While living with his wife and Children in Cape Town, his days aren't spent sad because he is confident that he served as oppressed people's voice.

Happy Person #2: Eva Peron

Eva Peron, the 2nd wife of the Argentine president Juan Peron, was a jolly fellow as she made a difference in the lives of the working class Argentines. She ran charities, supervised government agencies in labor and health, and initiated the Female Peronist Party, the first large-scale group that championed women's suffrage.

Happy Person #3: Mother Teresa

After having founded organizations that arranged hospices for people with HIV, leprosy, and tuberculosis, Mother Teresa discovered happiness in serving others. For her, selflessness nurtures good karma and seeing the positive effects of her actions is priceless. As she dedicated her life to charity work, she proclaimed that she belongs to the world.

Why Would Kindness Make You Happy?

Kindness will make you happy as it lets you discover inner peace. It allows you to sort things out while showing you a picture of yourself as a good person. Especially if you're the type who is usually apathetic, kindness will benefit you. It gives you the idea that you are bigger than you imagined yourself to be. Also, you have to admit that if you were the one in need, you'll be made happy if someone did the same to you.

Ten Acts of Kindness You Can Do

1. Buy lunch for a homeless person.

2. Do a week's worth of laundry for a family member.

3. Donate blood.

4. Gather old clothes and give it to the less fortunate.

5. Give a waiter a generous tip.

6. Listen intently to someone's problems.

7. Leave extra money on a vending machine.

8. Pay the toll fee for the vehicle-owner behind you.

9. Run errands for a neighbor.

10. Visit an orphanage and bring with you some goodies.

Thanks for Previewing My Exciting Book Entitled:

"Happiness! Secrets From The Happiest People On Earth"

To purchase this book, simply go to the Amazon Kindle store and simply search:

"HAPPINESS"

Then just scroll down until you see my book. You will know it is mine because you will see my name "Mia Conrad" underneath the title.

Alternatively, you can visit my author page on Amazon to see this book and other work I have done. Thanks so much, and please don't forget your free bonuses

DON'T LEAVE YET! - CHECK OUT YOUR FREE BONUSES BELOW!

Free Bonus Offer: Get Free Access To The PotentialRise.com VIP Newsletter!

Once you enter your email address you will immediately get free access to this awesome newsletter!

But wait, right now if you join now for free you will also get free access to the "LIMITLESS ENERGY" free EBook!

To claim both your FREE VIP NEWSLETTER MEMBERSHIP and your FREE BONUS Ebook on LIMITLESS ENERGY!

Just Go To:

www.PotentialRise.com